BREAST CANCER DIET BOOK FOR ADULT

ESSENTIAL NUTRITIONAL APPROACHES FOR ADULTS AND OPTIMIZING HEALTH AND WELLNESS THROUGH DIET IN BREAST CANCER MANAGEMENT AND PREVENTION

Sanucci hunkie

TABLE OF CONTENT

CHAPTER 1: THE BASICS OF BREAST CANCER 16
WHAT IS BREAST CANCER? 17
CHAPTER 2: THE ROLE OF NUTRITION IN CANCER PREVENTION 36
UNDERSTANDING CANCER FIGHTING NUTRIENTS...................36
CHAPTER 3: BUILDING A CANCER FIGHTING DIET 55
MACRONUTRIENTS AND MICRONUTRIENTS 55
CHAPTER 4: FOODS TO AVOID......................74
PROCESSED FOODS AND SUGARS..........74
CHAPTER 5: SPECIAL CONSIDERATIONS DURING TREATMENT 95
NUTRITION DURING CHEMOTHERAPY AND RADIATION 95

INTRODUCTION

Breast cancer is a profound and frequently life converting analysis that affects tens of millions of individuals worldwide. This ebook aims to empower adults, whether they're newly identified, in treatment, or in remission, with the information and tools to make informed dietary choices. By imparting scientifically sponsored facts and realistic steering, we are hoping to help your adventure in the direction of better fitness and stepped forward outcomes.

UNDERSTANDING BREAST CANCER

Breast cancer is the maximum common most cancers among women globally, with a sizable wide variety of cases identified every yr. It can arise in both women and men, although it is far extra commonplace in ladies. Understanding the nature of breast most cancers, inclusive of its diverse types and ranges, is critical for all of us suffering from this ailment. Knowledge is electricity, and through instructing yourself about breast cancer, you could take proactive steps closer to coping with your health.

IMPORTANCE OF DIET IN BREAST CANCER

Prevention and Management

While there may be no single cause of breast most cancers, research has proven that weight reduction plan plays a critical position in each the prevention and control of this sickness. Certain foods and nutritional patterns can impact your danger of developing breast cancer, as well as your potential to deal with treatment and healing. This ebook will explore the connections among food regimen and breast most cancers, imparting practical advice on how to nourish your frame at some point of each section of your adventure.

Scientific Insights: Clear causes of the modern day studies on weight reduction plan and breast most cancers.

Dietary Guidelines: Practical advice on what to eat and what to avoid to aid your fitness.

Meal Plans and Recipes: Nutritious and scrumptious recipes designed to meet your dietary desires.

Personal Stories: Inspiring memories from breast most cancers survivors who have benefited from dietary modifications.

Resources and Support: Information on extra sources, together with guide businesses and expert businesses.

THE ROLE OF DIET IN BREAST CANCER PREVENTION

Diet is a modifiable chance component that can significantly have an effect on your usual health and your chance of growing breast cancer. Scientific research has recognized several nutritional styles and specific ingredients which can help lessen the risk of breast most cancers.

Antioxidant Rich Foods: Foods excessive in antioxidants, such as fruits and greens, can assist guard cells from harm. Antioxidants like nutrients C and E, carotenoids, and flavonoid neutralize unfastened radicals, which are risky molecules that could reason cell harm and contribute to cancer improvement.

Fiber Rich Diets: Consuming a eating regimen excessive in nutritional fiber, determined in whole grains, culmination, veggies, and legumes, can assist reduce the risk of breast cancer. Fiber enables alter hormones, which includes estrogen, that could play a position in breast most cancers development.

Healthy Fats: Incorporating healthy fats, along with omega three fatty acids discovered in fish, flax seeds, and walnuts, could have anti inflammatory consequences and may lessen breast cancer risk. Avoiding trans fats and restricting saturated fat is likewise endorsed.

Phytoestrogens: Found in ingredients like soy products, flaxseeds, and complete grains, phytoestrogens are plant compounds that can mimic or modulate the body's estrogen tiers. Consuming those meals in moderation may have protecting results towards breast most cancers.

Cruciferous Vegetables: Vegetables like broccoli, cauliflower, and Brussels sprouts comprise compounds like sulforaphane and indolethreecarbinol, which have been proven to have anticancer homes.

Diet and Breast Cancer Management
For those identified with breast cancer, weight loss plan can play a critical role in

assisting remedy and improving first rate of lifestyles.

Maintaining a Healthy Weight: Obesity is associated with an accelerated danger of breast cancer recurrence and decreased survival charges. A balanced food regimen that promotes a healthy weight can enhance treatment consequences and average health.

Nutrient Dense Foods: During remedy, it is vital to devour nutrient dense foods that offer good enough nutrients, minerals, and electricity. Treatments like chemotherapy and radiation can increase dietary wishes and result in aspect outcomes that have an effect on appetite and nutrient absorption.

Managing Side Effects: Certain meals can assist manage aspect outcomes of most cancers remedy, which includes nausea, fatigue, and digestive troubles. For example, ginger can assist alleviate nausea, even as small, frequent food may help with appetite loss.

Supporting Immune Function: A weightreduction plan wealthy in vitamins and minerals, specifically those who guide immune function, consisting of diet C, nutrition D, and zinc, can assist the frame fight infections and recover extra efficiently from treatment.

Reducing Inflammation: Chronic infection is related to most cancers progression. Anti inflammatory ingredients, consisting of those rich in omega three fatty acids, antioxidants, and phytonutrients, can assist reduce irritation inside the frame.

Long Term Health and Survivorship
For breast most cancers survivors, maintaining a wholesome diet is important for longtime period health and decreasing the risk of recurrence. Key techniques include:

Balanced Diet: A food regimen that consists of lots of end result, veggies, whole grains, lean proteins, and healthful fat helps typical health and well being.

Physical Activity: Combining a healthy eating regimen with everyday bodily interest can help maintain a healthy weight and enhance overall health.

Regular Monitoring: Regular comply withdrawal healthcare providers, consisting of nutritionists and dietitians, can assist survivors live on the right track with their nutritional desires and deal with any nutritional deficiencies.

Explanation of the way weight loss plan can effect breast most cancers chance and restoration

Explanation of How Diet Can Impact Breast Cancer Risk and Recovery

Impact of Diet on Breast Cancer Risk

Diet is a critical aspect that could affect the chance of growing breast cancer.

1. Hormone Regulation:

- Estrogen Levels: Certain dietary selections can have an effect on estrogen tiers within the frame. High degrees of estrogen were related to an elevated hazard of hormone receptor wonderful breast cancer. Diets wealthy in fiber can help reduce estrogen tiers by means of selling the excretion of estrogen within the digestive tract.

- Phytoestrogens: Foods containing phytoestrogens, which includes soy merchandise, will have a mild estrogenic impact, which may also help alter the body's herbal estrogen ranges and decrease breast most cancers threat.

2. Inflammation and Oxidative Stress:

- AntioxidantRich Foods: Diets high in fruits and greens offer antioxidants that assist neutralize loose radicals, reducing oxidative strain and mobile damage that can result in cancer.

- Anti Inflammatory Foods: Consuming ingredients with anti inflammatory properties, along with fatty fish (rich in omega3 fatty acids), nuts, seeds, and olive oil, can decrease continual infection, which is associated with cancer development.

3. Body Weight and Obesity:

- Caloric Intake: A balanced food regimen that continues a wholesome body weight is vital, as obesity is a vast chance component for breast cancer. Excess frame fat can boom estrogen ranges and sell irritation, both of which contribute to breast cancer hazard.

- Nutrient Dense Foods: Choosing nutrient dense meals over high calorie, low nutrient options can assist manage weight and offer essential vitamins for ordinary health.

4. Dietary Patterns:

- Mediterranean Diet: This eating regimen emphasizes end result, vegetables, entire grains, legumes, nuts, seeds, and olive oil, with slight fish and rooster consumption. It is associated with a lower chance of breast most cancers because of its anti inflammatory and antioxidant homes.

- Plant Based Diets: Diets wealthy in plant based totally meals and low in red and processed meats were connected to a reduced hazard of breast cancer.

IMPACT OF DIET ON BREAST
CANCER RECOVERY

For people recognized with breast most cancers, food plan performs a giant function in helping remedy and restoration.

1. Nutrient Support During Treatment:

- High Quality Protein: Adequate protein intake is crucial for tissue repair and immune feature, specifically throughout chemotherapy and radiation. Sources encompass lean meats, fish, eggs, dairy, legumes, and nuts.

- Vitamins and Minerals: Consuming a variety of fruits and veggies ensures an adequate consumption of important nutrients and minerals, which aid typical fitness and help mitigate remedy side results.

2. Managing Treatment Side Effects:

Nausea and Vomiting: Foods like ginger, crackers, and small, common food can help manage nausea. Staying hydrated with clean fluids and herbal teas is likewise beneficial.

Fatigue: Nutrient dense meals and adequate hydration can assist combat remedy associated fatigue. Complex carbohydrates and lean proteins provide sustained power.

3. Immune System Support:

- Immune Boosting Foods: Foods rich in nutrients A, C, D, E, and zinc, together with citrus culmination, leafy veggies, nuts, seeds, and fortified dairy merchandise, support the immune device.

- Probiotics: Fermented foods like yogurt, kefir, sauerkraut, and kimchi promote intestine fitness, that's closely linked to immune function.

4. Reducing Recurrence Risk:

- Balanced Diet: Maintaining a balanced weightreduction plan with an emphasis on plant based totally foods, wholesome fat, and lean proteins can help reduce the risk of most cancers recurrence.

- Healthy Lifestyle: Combining a wholesome weight loss plan with regular bodily hobby, stress control, and keeping off smoking and immoderate alcohol consumption contributes to overall health and decreases recurrence hazard.

5. Long Term Health:

- Cardiovascular Health: Some breast most cancers treatments can have an effect on heart fitness. A coronary heart healthy eating regimen that includes complete grains, fruits, vegetables, lean proteins, and healthy fats can assist mitigate these effects.

CHAPTER 1: THE BASICS OF BREAST CANCER

WHAT IS BREAST CANCER?

Definition and Types of Breast Cancer
Breast cancer is a kind of cancer that begins in the cells of the breast. It happens whilst cells within the breast develop uncontrollably and shape a tumor. These cancerous cells can invade surrounding tissues and spread to different parts of the frame (metastasize). Breast cancer commonly affects women but can also arise in guys.

TYPES OF BREAST CANCER
Breast cancer is assessed based totally on in which it originates inside the breast tissue and the characteristics of the cancer cells.

1. Ductal Carcinoma In Situ (DCIS)

- Definition: DCIS is a noninvasive breast most cancers in which atypical cells are found inside the lining of a breast duct but have not spread outdoor the duct.

- Characteristics: Considered the earliest shape of breast most cancers, DCIS is highly treatable and has a low risk of becoming invasive if detected early.

2. Invasive Ductal Carcinoma (IDC)

Definition: IDC is the maximum not unusual form of breast most cancers, accounting for approximately 80% of all instances. It begins within the ducts after which invades nearby tissue within the breast.

Characteristics: IDC can unfold to different components of the body via the lymphatic system and bloodstream.

3. Invasive Lobular Carcinoma (ILC)

Definition: ILC starts off evolved inside the lobules (milk producing glands) of the breast and might spread to close by tissues and other components of the body.

Characteristics: ILC is the second most commonplace type of invasive breast cancer, making up approximately 1015% of cases.

4. Triple Negative Breast Cancer

Definition: This type of breast most cancers lacks three commonplace receptors recognised to fuel most breast most cancers boom: estrogen receptors (ER), progesterone receptors (PR), and human epidermal increase component receptor 2 (HER2).

Characteristics: Triplenegative breast cancer is greater aggressive and hard to deal with because it does not reply to hormonal remedy or HER2centered treatments.

5. HER2Positive Breast Cancer

Definition: HER2advantageous breast most cancers has high tiers of the HER2 protein, which promotes the growth of cancer cells.

Characteristics: This kind tends to grow quicker however can be treated with capsules that mainly target the HER2 protein.

6. Hormone Receptor Positive Breast Cancer

Definition: These cancers have cells that include receptors for hormones like estrogen (ERfine) and/or progesterone (PReffective).

Characteristics: Hormone receptor wonderful cancers may be treated with hormonal therapies that block these hormones or decrease their stages in the body.

7. Inflammatory Breast Cancer (IBC)

Definition: IBC is a unprecedented and competitive form of breast most cancers that spreads fast, causing the breast to end up red, swollen, and warm.

Characteristics: IBC is frequently wrong for an infection because of its signs and symptoms and calls for spark off remedy.

8. Paget's Disease of the Nipple

Definition: This rare form of breast cancer starts off evolved within the ducts of the nipple and extends to the nipple's floor and areola.

Characteristics: Symptoms consist of redness, itching, and a burning sensation in the nipple place, regularly with discharge.

RISK FACTORS FOR BREAST CANCER

Understanding the risk elements for breast most cancers can help people take preventive measures and make informed choices approximately their fitness. While a few risk elements are past manage, others may be managed thru way of life changes.

Non Modifiable Risk Factors

1. Gender

Women are at a considerably better hazard of developing breast most cancers in comparison to guys.

2. Age

The threat of breast most cancers increases with age, with maximum instances recognized in girls over 50.

3. Genetic Mutations

Inherited mutations in genes along with BRCA1 and BRCA2 significantly boom the chance of breast most cancers. Other genetic mutations may additionally make contributions to multiplied threat.

4. Family History

Having near family (consisting of a mother, sister, or daughter) with breast cancer increases an man or woman's risk, mainly if the relative was identified at a young age.

5. Personal History of Breast Cancer

Individuals who have had breast most cancers are at a better danger of growing a new most cancers within the other breast or some other a part of the identical breast.

6. Race and Ethnicity

White ladies are slightly more likely to develop breast cancer than African American, Hispanic, and Asian girls. However, African American girls are much more likely to develop competitive, early onset breast cancer.

7. Dense Breast Tissue

Women with dense breast tissue have a higher hazard of breast most cancers and can require additional screening strategies.

8. Previous Radiation Therapy

Individuals who have had radiation therapy to the chest, specifically earlier than age 30, are at extended danger.

GENETIC AND WAY OF LIFE ELEMENTS contributing to breast most cancers

Genetic and Lifestyle Factors Contributing to Breast Cancer

GENETIC FACTORS

1. Inherited Gene Mutations

- BRCA1 and BRCA2 Mutations: Mutations inside the BRCA1 and BRCA2 genes extensively boom the danger of breast cancer. These genes usually assist restore DNA damage, but whilst mutated, they fail to feature well, main to increased cancer hazard.

- Other Genetic Mutations: Mutations in genes such as TP53, PTEN, and PALB2 additionally make a contribution to higher breast cancer chance. These mutations are much less common however nevertheless play a good sized function in hereditary breast most cancers.

2. Family History

Having close relatives (including a mother, sister, or daughter) with breast cancer, mainly in the event that they were recognized at a young age, will increase an person's chance. The danger is better if a couple of circle of relatives members are affected or if there may be a regarded genetic mutation in the own family.

3. Personal History of Breast Cancer

Individuals who've had breast most cancers are at a better chance of growing new cancer inside the other breast or another part of the identical breast.

4. Ethnicity

Certain genetic mutations, which includes BRCA1 and BRCA2, are more common in unique ethnic organizations, such as

Ashkenazi Jewish ladies, who've a better occurrence of those mutations.

LIFESTYLE FACTORS

1. Diet and Nutrition

- High Fat Diet: Diets excessive in saturated fats and trans fat may also increase breast cancer hazard. Conversely, diets rich in end result, veggies, and whole grains are associated with a decrease danger.

- Alcohol Consumption: Regular consumption of alcohol will increase the threat of breast cancer. Even moderate ingesting can raise the chance.

- Obesity: Being obese or obese, in particular after menopause, will increase the hazard because of better degrees of estrogen produced through fats tissue.

2. Physical Activity

Regular bodily interest helps preserve a healthy weight and has been proven to lessen breast cancer hazard. Exercise also can assist adjust hormone stages and enhance immune function.

3. Reproductive and Hormonal Factors

- Early Menstruation and Late Menopause: Early onset of menstruation (before age 12) and late menopause (after age 55) extend the lifetime exposure to estrogen, increasing breast most cancers threat.

- Childbearing and Breastfeeding: Having the first infant at a later age or not having kids at all can boom risk. Breastfeeding, particularly for extra extended duration, can reduce the chance.

4. Hormone Replacement Therapy (HRT)

Longtime period use of hormone substitute remedy, particularly combined estrogen progesterone remedy, will increase the hazard of breast most cancers. The risk decreases once the therapy is stopped.

5. Exposure to Radiation

Previous exposure to radiation remedy, especially to the chest location and at a younger age, will increase the danger of growing breast most cancers later in existence.

6. Smoking

Smoking, especially lengthy time period smoking and smoking at a young age, is related to an accelerated risk of breast cancer. It may make contributions to more aggressive sorts of the ailment.

7. Environmental Factors

Exposure to positive chemical substances and environmental pollutants, which include the ones located in a few plastics and insecticides, may additionally boom breast most cancers hazard. Ongoing research continues to research those hyperlinks.

8. Stress and Psychological Factors

While the direct link between pressure and breast cancer continues to be beneath investigation, continual stress may additionally result in behaviors (e.G., bad weight loss plan, lack of exercising, smoking) that boom hazard.

SYMPTOMS AND DIAGNOSIS OF BREAST CANCER

Breast most cancers can present with various symptoms, however it's vital to word that early level breast cancer might not constantly purpose important symptoms. Regular screening mammograms are crucial for early detection.

1. Lump or Thickening

A lump or thickening inside the breast or underarm area is regularly the first major symptom of breast cancer. Not all lumps are cancerous, but any new lump must be evaluated by a healthcare professional.

2. Changes in Breast Size or Shape

Changes inside the length, shape, or look of the breast, such as swelling, dimpling, or puckering of the pores and skin, may imply breast cancer.

3. Changes inside the Skin

Redness, rash, or scaling of the breast pores and skin, mainly around the nipple, may be symptoms of breast most cancers.

4. Nipple Changes

Changes inside the nipple, which includes inversion (pulling inward), flattening, or discharge (apart from breast milk), ought to be evaluated.

5. Pain

While breast cancer itself is normally no longer painful within the early stages, chronic breast pain or soreness that does not leave with the menstrual cycle or varies in depth ought to be checked by using a doctor.

6. Swelling

Swelling or lumps inside the lymph nodes inside the armpit or around the collarbone can be a sign that breast most cancers has spread.

TREATMENT OPTIONS FOR BREAST CANCER

Treatment for breast most cancers varies relying on the type and level of the most cancers, in addition to different person factors which includes universal fitness and preferences. The number one treatment options encompass:

SURGERY

1. Lumpectomy (Breast preserving surgical procedure)

Description: Removal of the tumor and a small margin of surrounding wholesome tissue. It goals to preserve the breast as tons as possible.

Indication: Typically used for early degree breast cancer in which the tumor is small and localized.

2. Mastectomy

Description: Surgical removal of the entire breast tissue, once in a while consisting of the nipple and areola.

Types:

- Simple or Total Mastectomy: Removal of the complete breast tissue but no longer the lymph nodes.

- Modified Radical Mastectomy: Removal of the whole breast tissue and some of the lymph nodes beneath the arm.

- Radical Mastectomy: Rarely carried out nowadays; elimination of the breast tissue, lymph nodes below the arm, and chest wall muscle groups.

RADIATION THERAPY

Description: Uses high electricity rays (along with Xrays or protons) to kill cancer cells. It can be used after surgical treatment (breast protecting surgical procedure or mastectomy) to wreck last most cancers cells or reduce the danger of recurrence.

Indication: Often encouraged for sufferers with early stage breast cancer to reduce the chance of local recurrence.

CHEMOTHERAPY

Description: Treatment with capsules that kill cancer cells or forestall them from developing. It may be given intravenously or orally.

Indication: Used in diverse conditions, inclusive of after surgery to lessen the threat of most cancers recurrence, earlier than surgical treatment to shrink tumors (neoadjuvant therapy), or for superiorstage breast cancer to sluggish cancer increase.

HORMONE THERAPY

Description: Blocks hormones or lowers their ranges in the body to stop or slow the growth of hormone receptor high quality breast cancers.

Indication: Typically used for hormone receptor fantastic breast cancers, which rely upon hormones (estrogen and/or progesterone) to grow.

TARGETED THERAPY

Description: Uses drugs that focus on particular characteristics of cancer cells, consisting of HER2advantageous breast cancers.

Indication: Used in combination with different treatments to mainly goal cancer cells at the same time as minimizing harm to regular cells.

Description: Uses capsules that help the
immune system understand and attack
cancer cells.

Indication: Being studied in clinical trials
for breast most cancers remedy, mainly in
triple poor breast cancers.

CLINICAL TRIALS

Description: Research studies that take a
look at new treatments or treatment mixtures.
They provide get entry to to probably
promising remedies that aren't but widely to
be had.

SUPPORTIVE CARE

Description: Includes remedies and
treatment plans that assist manage signs and
symptoms and aspect effects of breast
cancer remedy, consisting of pain
management, nutrition support, and
psychological guide.

CHAPTER 2: THE ROLE OF NUTRITION IN CANCER PREVENTION

UNDERSTANDING CANCER FIGHTING NUTRIENTS

ANTIOXIDANTS, PHYTOCHEMICALS, AND DIFFERENT KEY NUTRIENTS

Antioxidants, Phytochemicals, and Other Key Nutrients in Breast Cancer Prevention and Management

ANTIOXIDANTS

1. Vitamin C

Source: Citrus culmination (oranges, grapefruits), strawberries, kiwi, bell peppers, broccoli.

Role: Acts as a powerful antioxidant, defensive cells from oxidative damage which could cause cancer.

2. Vitamin E

Source: Nuts (almonds, hazelnuts), seeds (sunflower seeds, flaxseeds), spinach, broccoli.

Role: Protects cells from oxidative strain and helps immune function.

3. BetaCarotene

Source: Carrots, candy potatoes, spinach, kale, apricots.

Role: Converts to nutrition A within the body, supports immune function, and acts as an antioxidant.

4. Selenium

Source: Brazil nuts, seafood (oysters, shrimp), complete grains (brown rice, wheat germ), sunflower seeds.

Role: Acts as a co factor for antioxidant enzymes and allows protect in opposition to oxidative harm.

Phytochemicals

1. Flavonoids

Source: Berries (blueberries, strawberries), citrus end result, onions, tea (inexperienced and black tea).

Role: Have antioxidant and anti inflammatory homes, doubtlessly reducing most cancers hazard.

2. Isoflavones

Source: Soybeans and soy merchandise (tofu, soy milk), chickpeas, lentils.

Role: Phytoestrogens which can have protective results in opposition to hormone associated cancers like breast most cancers.

3. Indoles and Glucosinolates

Source: Cruciferous vegetables (broccoli, cauliflower, Brussels sprouts), cabbage.

Role: Have potential anticancer consequences, together with the ability to regulate estrogen metabolism.

Other Key Nutrients

1. Omega three Fatty Acids

Source: Fatty fish (salmon, mackerel), flaxseeds, chia seeds, walnuts.

Role: Have anti inflammatory results and can lessen most cancers hazard and aid common cardiovascular health.

2. Fiber

Source: Whole grains (oats, brown rice), end result (apples, berries), vegetables (carrots, broccoli).

Role: Aids in digestion, helps modify hormones like estrogen, and can decrease breast cancer risk.

3. Cruciferous Vegetables

Source: Broccoli, cauliflower, Brussels sprouts, kale.

Role: Contain compounds like sulforaphane and indolethreecarbinol, which have been studied for their capacity most cancers preventive homes.

4. Probiotics

Source: Yogurt with live cultures, kefir, sauerkraut, kimchi.

Role: Support gut fitness and may enhance immune feature, probably impacting standard health and cancer threat.

IMPORTANCE IN BREAST CANCER PREVENTION AND MANAGEMENT

- Antioxidants and photochemical assist neutralize unfastened radicals and decrease oxidative pressure, that may damage cells and make a contribution to cancer improvement.

- Omega three fatty acids and a food plan wealthy in fiber and cruciferous vegetables may assist alter hormone tiers and support immune feature, decreasing breast cancer chance.

- Including probiotics may sell a wholesome gut microbiome, which

performs a function in immune
characteristic and standard health.

FOODS THAT PREVENT CANCER

Foods which can be frequently related to most cancers prevention normally comprise particular vitamins, antioxidants, and phytochemicals that help usual health and may help reduce the danger of numerous forms of most cancers, consisting of breast most cancers.

1. Fruits and Vegetables

Berries: Blueberries, strawberries, raspberries are rich in antioxidants like anthocyanins and diet C.

Cruciferous Vegetables: Broccoli, cauliflower, Brussels sprouts comprise sulforaphane and indole3carbinol, which may also have most cancers protective homes.

Leafy Greens: Spinach, kale, Swiss chard are wealthy in vitamins, minerals, and phytochemicals.

Tomatoes: Rich in lycopene, a effective antioxidant.

Citrus Fruits: Oranges, grapefruits, lemons are high in vitamin C and flavonoids.

2. Whole Grains

Oats: Rich in fiber and antioxidants.

Brown Rice: Contains fiber, nutrients, and minerals.

Quinoa: High in protein, fiber, and diverse vitamins.

3. Legumes and Beans

Beans: Black beans, kidney beans, lentils are high in fiber, protein, and antioxidants.

Soy Products: Tofu, tempeh, soy milk comprise phytoestrogens (isoflavones) which could have protecting consequences.

4. Nuts and Seeds

Almonds: Rich in diet E and healthy fat.

Walnuts: High in omega3 fatty acids.

Flaxseeds and Chia Seeds: Good sources of omegathree fatty acids and fiber.

5. Healthy Fats

Olive Oil: Contains monounsaturated fats and antioxidants.

Avocados: Rich in wholesome fats, fiber, and antioxidants.

6. Fish

Fatty Fish: Salmon, mackerel, sardines are high in omega3 fatty acids.

7. Herbs and Spices

Turmeric: Contains curcumin, a potent anti inflammatory compound.

Garlic: Contains sulfur compounds with potential anticancer houses.

Ginger: Has antioxidant and anti inflammatory consequences.

8. Green Tea

Green Tea: Contains polyphenols (catechins) with antioxidant properties.

9. Probiotic Foods

Yogurt: Contains beneficial probiotics that help intestine fitness.

10. Dark Chocolate

Dark Chocolate: High in antioxidants and flavonoids.

HOW THEY HELP PREVENT CANCER

Antioxidants: Protect cells from harm due to unfastened radicals, lowering the risk of most cancers.

Phytochemicals: Plant compounds with capability anticancer homes, such as anti inflammatory and antioxidant consequences.

Fiber: Aids in digestion, facilitates alter hormones, and helps typical intestine health, which might also effect most cancers threat.

Healthy Fats: Omega3 fatty acids have anti inflammatory homes that may lessen most cancers threat.

Probiotics: Support a healthful gut microbiome, which plays a function in immune characteristic and inflammation, POTENTIALLY IMPACTING CANCER PREVENTION.

List of unique foods with cancer preventive houses

1. Berries

Blueberries, Strawberries, Raspberries

Beneficial Compounds: Anthocyanins, diet C, fiber

2. Cruciferous Vegetables

Broccoli, Cauliflower, Brussels Sprouts

Beneficial Compounds: Sulforaphane, indolethreecarbinol, fiber

3. Leafy Greens

Spinach, Kale, Swiss Chard

Beneficial Compounds: Vitamins (A, C, K), folate, fiber, antioxidants

4. Tomatoes

Beneficial Compounds: Lycopene, diet C, potassium

5. Citrus Fruits

Oranges, Grapefruits, Lemons

Beneficial Compounds: Vitamin C, flavonoids, fiber

6. Garlic

Beneficial Compounds: Allicin, sulfur compounds

7. Turmeric

Beneficial Compounds: Curcumin (energetic compound), antioxidants

8. Green Tea

Beneficial Compounds: Catechins (inclusive of EGCG), antioxidants

9. Berries

Blueberries, Strawberries, Raspberries

Beneficial Compounds: Anthocyanins, diet C, fiber

10. Nuts and Seeds

Almonds, Walnuts, Flaxseeds

Beneficial Compounds: Omegathree fatty acids, diet E, fiber

11. Whole Grains

Oats, Brown Rice, Quinoa

Beneficial Compounds: Fiber, antioxidants, vitamins (B complicated)

12. Legumes and Beans

Black Beans, Lentils, Chickpeas

Beneficial Compounds: Fiber, protein, antioxidants

13. Soy Products

Tofu, Tempeh, Soy Milk

Beneficial Compounds: Isoflavones (phytoestrogens), protein, fiber

14. Fish

Salmon, Mackerel, Sardines

Beneficial Compounds: Omegathree fatty acids, protein

15. Olive Oil

Beneficial Compounds: Monounsaturated fats, antioxidants

16. Yogurt

Beneficial Compounds: Probiotics, calcium, protein

17. Dark Chocolate (70% or higher cocoa content material)

Beneficial Compounds: Flavonoids, antioxidants

DIETARY PATTERNS FOR CANCER PREVENTION

When it comes to cancer prevention, nutritional patterns that emphasize whole ingredients, plant based totally resources of vitamins, and a balanced consumption of key vitamins have proven promise.

1. Mediterranean Diet

Key Features:

Rich in culmination, veggies, whole grains, nuts, and seeds.

Includes olive oil as the number one source of fats.

Moderate consumption of fish, hen, and dairy merchandise.

Red wine consumed moderately (nonobligatory).

Limited intake of purple and processed meats.

Potential Benefits:

- High in antioxidants and phytochemicals which could guard towards oxidative pressure and inflammation.

- Rich in fiber, which helps digestive fitness and can assist alter hormone tiers.

- Healthy fats from olive oil and nuts may additionally have anti inflammatory houses.

2. Plant Based Diet

Key Features:

Emphasis on culmination, vegetables, complete grains, legumes, nuts, and seeds.

Minimal or no animal products, along with meat and dairy.

Includes resources of plant based totally proteins such as tofu, tempeh, and beans.

Potential Benefits:

- High in fiber, vitamins, and minerals, which aid typical fitness and immune characteristic.

- Low in saturated fats and cholesterol, which may also reduce inflammation and aid heart fitness.

- Phytochemicals and antioxidants determined in plant meals may additionally have protecting outcomes against cancer.

3. DASH Diet (Dietary Approaches to Stop Hypertension)

Key Features:

- Emphasizes culmination, veggies, whole grains, and lean proteins.

- Limits sodium intake and promotes ingredients rich in potassium, calcium, and magnesium.

- Encourages slight consumption of dairy merchandise and nuts.

Potential Benefits:

- Supports heart health and can assist reduce the danger of high blood pressure and cardiovascular ailment.

- Rich in antioxidants and phytochemicals from fruits and vegetables.

- Emphasis on complete grains and coffeefat dairy products may also contribute to common health and cancer prevention.

4. AntiInflammatory Diet

Key Features:

- Focuses on ingredients that lessen irritation within the frame, together with fruits, veggies, whole grains, nuts, fatty fish, and wholesome fats (e.G., olive oil).

- Limits or avoids processed meals, sugary drinks, and red and processed meats.

- Includes herbs and spices known for his or her anti inflammatory houses, which includes turmeric and ginger.

Potential Benefits:

Reduces persistent inflammation, that's related to improved most cancers hazard.

Provides a whole lot of vitamins and antioxidants that help immune characteristic and typical fitness.

General Guidelines for Cancer Prevention:

Limit Red and Processed Meats: Reduce intake of red meats (beef, beef) and processed meats (sausages, bacon) which can be connected to better cancer hazard, mainly colorectal most cancers.

Moderate Alcohol Consumption: Limit alcohol intake, as immoderate alcohol consumption is connected to elevated hazard of several cancers, inclusive of breast most cancers.

Maintain a Healthy Weight: Aim for a healthy frame weight through a balanced food regimen and regular physical activity. Obesity is associated with multiplied risk of several cancers.

Stay Hydrated: Drink plenty of water and restriction sugary beverages and liquids excessive in energy.

Limit Sugary and Processed Foods: Reduce consumption of foods excessive in brought sugars, subtle grains, and unhealthy fats.

Be Mindful of Food Preparation: Avoid charred or burnt meals, as cooking meats at high temperatures can produce carcinogenic compounds.

CHAPTER 3: BUILDING A CANCER FIGHTING DIET

MACRONUTRIENTS AND MICRONUTRIENTS

IMPORTANCE OF BALANCED MACRONUTRIENTS (CARBOHYDRATES, PROTEINS, FATS)

Balanced macronutrients play a vital function in retaining typical health and properlybeing.

1. Energy Source and Metabolism

- Carbohydrates: Are the body's primary and most efficient source of strength. They are damaged down into glucose, which fuels cells, in particular the ones in the mind and muscle tissues.

- Proteins: Essential for building and repairing tissues, which includes muscle tissues, organs, and immune cells. They additionally play a position in enzyme and hormone manufacturing.

- Fats: Provide a focused supply of electricity and assist inside the absorption of fat soluble nutrients (A, D, E, K). They additionally contribute to mobile membrane structure and feature.

2. Nutrient Absorption and Transport

- Carbohydrates: Provide fiber, which aids in digestion and allows adjust blood sugar stages. Some carbohydrates additionally act as prebiotics, assisting gut fitness.

- Proteins: Assist in nutrient shipping and help keep fluid balance within the frame. They are also worried within the synthesis of antibodies and enzymes.

- Fats: Essential for the absorption of fat soluble nutrients (A, D, E, K) and positive phytochemicals. They also assist maintain pores and skin and hair fitness.

3. Hormone Regulation

- Carbohydrates: Influence insulin degrees, which adjust blood sugar and electricity metabolism.

- Proteins: Are involved in the manufacturing of hormones, such as insulin and growth hormone.

- Fats: Play a function in hormone manufacturing and regulation, along with sex hormones like estrogen and testosterone.

4. Cell Structure and Function

Carbohydrates: Are necessary for the synthesis of glycoproteins and glycolipids, that are components of cell membranes.

Proteins: Form the structure of cells, tissues, and organs, and are necessary to the feature of enzymes and delivery proteins.

Fats: Contribute to the structure and feature of mobile membranes, nerve cells, and myelin sheaths.

5. Maintaining Healthy Weight and Body Composition

- Balanced Intake: Helps modify appetite and promotes satiety, lowering the chance of overeating or immoderate snacking.

- Proteins: Are mainly satiating, supporting to preserve lean muscle tissues for the duration of weight reduction or preservation levels.

- Fats: Provide a sense of fullness and pleasure, that can save you cravings and help longtime period dietary adherence.

Practical Tips for Achieving Balanced Macronutrients:

Include Variety: Consume a variety of entire ingredients to make certain a balanced

consumption of carbohydrates, proteins, and
fat.

 Portion Control: Be mindful of component
sizes to keep away from over consumption
of any single macronutrient.

- Focus on Whole Foods: Prioritize entire
  grains, lean proteins, healthy fats,
  culmination, and greens over processed
  and sugary foods.

- Consider Individual Needs: Adjust
  macronutrient ratios primarily based on
  character health goals, interest ranges,
  and metabolic needs.

- Stay Hydrated: Drink masses of water
  during the day to help digestion and
  nutrient absorption.

- Key nutrients and minerals for breast
  fitness

Maintaining premiere breast fitness entails
making sure adequate consumption of
particular nutrients and minerals that help

average health and may have unique blessings for breast tissue.

KEY VITAMINS FOR BREAST HEALTH

1. Vitamin D

- Role: Helps alter cellular increase and differentiation. Adequate diet D ranges may additionally lessen breast most cancers hazard and help common breast health.

- Sources: Sunlight exposure (UVB rays), fatty fish (salmon, mackerel), fortified dairy merchandise, egg yolks.

2. Vitamin A

Role: Essential for preserving wholesome epithelial tissues, inclusive of breast tissue. It also acts as an antioxidant, protective cells from harm.

Sources: Liver, sweet potatoes, carrots, spinach, kale, dairy products.

3. Vitamin E

- Role: Acts as an antioxidant, protecting cellular membranes and DNA from damage. It might also help lessen oxidative pressure in breast tissue.

- Sources: Nuts (especially almonds), seeds (sunflower seeds), spinach, broccoli, avocado.

4. Vitamin C

Role: Essential for collagen synthesis and antioxidant protection. It might also help shield against oxidative strain and aid immune feature.

Sources: Citrus end result (oranges, grapefruits), strawberries, kiwi, bell peppers, broccoli.

KEY MINERALS FOR BREAST HEALTH

1. Calcium

Role: Essential for bone health and muscle function. Adequate calcium intake may reduce the chance of breast cancer and aid normal breast health.

Sources: Dairy merchandise (milk, yogurt, cheese), leafy vegetables (kale, collard vegetables), fortified plant based totally milks.

2. Magnesium

- Role: Important for enzyme function, strength manufacturing, and muscle rest. It may additionally assist lessen breast cancer chance.

- Sources: Nuts (almonds, cashews), seeds (pumpkin seeds, sunflower seeds), entire grains, leafy veggies.

3. Selenium

Role: Acts as an antioxidant, protective cells from oxidative damage. It additionally supports immune feature and thyroid fitness.

Sources: Brazil nuts, seafood (oysters, shrimp), whole grains (brown rice, wheat germ), sunflower seeds.

4. Zinc

- Role: Essential for immune function, wound healing, and DNA synthesis. It may additionally assist regulate mobile growth and reduce breast cancer chance.

- Sources: Oysters, beef, hen, beans, nuts, whole grains.

OTHER NUTRIENTS FOR BREAST HEALTH

- Omega3 Fatty Acids: Found in fatty fish (salmon, sardines), flax seeds, and walnuts. They have anti inflammatory houses and may help lessen breast most cancers risk.

- Hydrogenates: Plant compounds observed in soybeans and legumes which could have shielding consequences towards hormone associated cancers like breast cancer.

SUPER FOODS FOR BREAST CANCER PREVENTION

Super foods, a term frequently used to explain nutrient dense meals with ability fitness advantages, can play a function in assisting usual fitness and probably reducing the threat of breast most cancers. While no unmarried meals can save you most cancers, incorporating a whole lot of super foods into a balanced weight reduction plan wealthy in culmination, greens, entire grains, and lean proteins can contribute to normal fitness and properly being.

1. Cruciferous Vegetables

Examples: Broccoli, Cauliflower, Brussels Sprouts, Kale

Benefits: Rich in sulforaphane and indolethreecarbinol, compounds that can have anticancer residences by way of promoting cleansing of carcinogens and regulating estrogen metabolism.

2. Berries

Examples: Blueberries, Strawberries, Raspberries

Benefits: High in antioxidants consisting of anthocyanins and vitamin C, which assist neutralize unfastened radicals and decrease oxidative stress that may result in cancer improvement.

3. Fatty Fish

Examples: Salmon, Mackerel, Sardines

Benefits: Rich in omega three fatty acids, which have anti inflammatory residences and can help reduce the chance of breast cancer by means of influencing cell tactics and reducing infection.

4. Turmeric

Benefits: Contains curcumin, a compound with mighty anti inflammatory and antioxidant houses. Curcumin might also inhibit most cancers mobile increase and help immune characteristic.

5. Green Tea

Benefits: Contains catechins, particularly epigallocatechin gallate (EGCG), which have antioxidant residences and may assist guard cells from harm that could cause cancer.

6. Tomatoes

Benefits: Rich in lycopene, a effective antioxidant which could lessen the threat of breast most cancers by using shielding cells from oxidative strain and inflammation.

7. Flaxseeds

Benefits: High in lignans, a sort of phytoestrogen which can have susceptible estrogenic properties. Flax seeds also offer omega3 fatty acids and fiber, which help typical fitness and can help modify hormone degrees.

8. Walnuts

Benefits: High in alphalinolenic acid (ALA), an omegathree fatty acid, as well as antioxidants and phytosterols. Walnuts may help lessen irritation and oxidative strain, potentially decreasing cancer risk.

9. Soy Products

Examples: Tofu, Edamame, Soy Milk

Benefits: Contain isoflavones, phytoestrogens that may have protective effects against hormonerelated cancers like breast most cancers. Research shows slight soy consumption is safe and may be beneficial.

10. Dark Leafy Greens

Examples: Spinach, Kale, Swiss Chard

Benefits: Rich in nutrients, minerals, and antioxidants that assist immune feature, reduce inflammation, and promote ordinary health.

Incorporating Super foods Into Your Diet

- **Diversity:** Aim to consist of a number of super foods to your meals and snacks to maximise nutrient intake and fitness blessings.

- **Balance:** Pair super foods with different nutrient dense foods to create balanced food that provide a wide variety of vitamins, minerals, and phytonutrients.

Moderation: While superfoods offer fitness benefits, moderation and range are key. No single food or institution of meals can replace a balanced weightreduction plan and healthy lifestyle.

DETAILED LISTING AND ADVANTAGES OF SUPER FOODS

1. Cruciferous Vegetables

Examples: Broccoli, Cauliflower, Brussels Sprouts, Kale, Cabbage

Benefits:

Sulforaphane: Supports detoxing processes inside the body and can help lessen cancer hazard by means of inhibiting tumor increase.

Indole3carbinol: Helps alter estrogen metabolism, potentially reducing the hazard of hormoneassociated cancers like breast most cancers.

High in Fiber: Supports digestion and intestine health, that is related to basic immunity and disease prevention.

2. Berries

Examples: Blueberries, Strawberries, Raspberries, Blackberries

Benefits:

Antioxidants (Anthocyanins, Vitamin C): Protect cells from oxidative pressure and inflammation, reducing the chance of persistent illnesses consisting of most cancers.

Fiber: Supports digestive health and helps alter blood sugar degrees.

3. Fatty Fish

Examples: Salmon, Mackerel, Sardines, Trout

Benefits:

Omegathree Fatty Acids (EPA, DHA): Have anti inflammatory houses which can lessen the chance of persistent illnesses like heart sickness and most cancers.

Protein: Provides vital amino acids for muscle restore and immune feature.

4. Turmeric

Benefits:

Curcumin: Potent antiinflammatory and antioxidant homes, may inhibit cancer cell increase and decrease inflammation for the duration of the body.

Supports Liver Health: Aids in detoxification methods and helps usual liver function.

5. Green Tea

Benefits:

Catechins (EGCG): Powerful antioxidants that assist protect cells from damage, reduce irritation, and may decrease the chance of positive cancers.

Boosts Metabolism: Supports weight management and typical cardiovascular fitness.

CREATING BALANCED MEALS

Creating balanced food includes combining exclusive meals corporations to make sure you get numerous nutrients that support usual fitness and nicely being.

Components of a Balanced Meal:

1. Protein

- Sources: Lean meats (chicken, turkey), fish, tofu, tempeh, beans, lentils, eggs, dairy products (yogurt, cheese).

Role: Builds and upkeep tissues, helps immune characteristic, and helps regulate hormones.

2. Carbohydrates

Sources: Whole grains (brown rice, quinoa, oats), starchy veggies (candy potatoes, corn), legumes, fruits.

Role: Provides energy, fiber for digestive health, and crucial vitamins and minerals.

3. Healthy Fats

Sources: Avocado, nuts (almonds, walnuts), seeds (chia seeds, flaxseeds), olive oil, fatty fish (salmon, mackerel).

Role: Supports brain function, hormone manufacturing, and absorbs fats soluble vitamins (A, D, E, K).

4. Vegetables

Examples: Leafy greens (spinach, kale), cruciferous veggies (broccoli, cauliflower), colorful vegetables (bell peppers, carrots).

Role: Provides nutrients, minerals, antioxidants, and fiber; supports immune function and universal health.

5. Fruits

Examples: Berries (blueberries, strawberries), citrus end result (oranges, grapefruits), apples, bananas.

Role: Supplies nutrients, antioxidants, and fiber; helps digestive health and affords herbal sweetness.

CHAPTER 4: FOODS TO AVOID

PROCESSED FOODS AND SUGARS

IMPACT OF PROCESSED INGREDIENTS AND HIGH SUGAR INTAKE ON MOST CANCERS THREAT

The impact of processed meals and high sugar consumption on cancer threat is a place of growing problem and research.

PROCESSED FOODS

1. High in Additives and Preservatives: Processed ingredients often comprise additives, preservatives, and synthetic substances which can have carcinogenic houses or make a contribution to oxidative strain within the frame.

2. Low in Nutrients: Many processed ingredients are low in critical nutrients including vitamins, minerals, and fiber,

which might be important for typical health and lowering cancer risk.

3. High in Unhealthy Fats and Sodium: Processed foods may be high in unhealthy fat (trans fat, saturated fat) and sodium, which are connected to inflammation, cardiovascular sickness, and potentially cancer.

4. Formation of Carcinogenic Compounds: Certain processing strategies, which include high temperature cooking (e.G., frying, grilling), can cause the formation of carcinogenic compounds like acrylamide and polycyclic aromatic hydrocarbons (PAHs).

Five. Impact on Gut Health: Processed meals may also negatively effect intestine microbiota composition, that is important for immune function and irritation regulation, probably affecting cancer chance.

HIGH SUGAR INTAKE

1. Promotes Inflammation: Excessive sugar consumption can lead to continual inflammation, which plays a function inside the improvement and progression of most cancers.

2. Increases Insulin Levels: High sugar intake can cause spikes in blood sugar ranges, leading to improved insulin production. Insulin is a growth issue that may sell cancer mobile proliferation.

3. Promotes Obesity: Sugary meals and drinks are caloriedense and might make contributions to weight benefit and weight problems, which might be threat elements for several kinds of most cancers, consisting of breast and colorectal most cancers.

4. Alters Hormone Levels: High sugar consumption can also disrupt hormone degrees, inclusive of insulin and sex hormones (e.G., estrogen), that may affect

cancer hazard, mainly hormone touchy cancers.

5. Feeds Cancer Cells: Cancer cells regularly have a higher call for for glucose (sugar) in comparison to normal cells, and a high sugar food regimen may also probably gas most cancers mobile increase and proliferation.

RECOMMENDATIONS

- Choose Whole Foods: Opt for entire, minimally processed foods inclusive of fruits, veggies, whole grains, lean proteins, and healthful fats.

- Limit Added Sugars: Reduce consumption of sugary drinks, snacks, and cakes. Pay interest to meals labels and pick out products with lower introduced sugar content.

- Moderate Processed Foods: Limit intake of processed meats, sugary cereals, snacks, and speedy meals. Instead, prioritize homemade food with clean ingredients.

- Focus on Nutrient Density: Select ingredients wealthy in vitamins, minerals, antioxidants, and fiber to help typical health and decrease cancer risk.

Maintain a Healthy Weight: Adopt a balanced diet and normal bodily pastime to gain and preserve a healthy weight, which could lower the hazard of weight problems associated cancers.

HARMFUL FATS AND RED MEATS

Harmful fat and purple meats can impact health negatively, in particular regarding cancer hazard and typical properly being.

HARMFUL FATS

1. Saturated Fats

- Sources: Found in animal products including beef, complete fat dairy merchandise (butter, cheese), and some plant oils (coconut oil, palm oil).

- Impact: Consuming high amounts of saturated fat is linked to accelerated LDL cholesterol levels, which could make a contribution to cardiovascular ailment. Some research advise a hyperlink among saturated fat and positive cancers, even though the proof isn't as strong as for cardiovascular sickness.

2. Trans Fats

- Sources: Primarily located in partially hydrogenated oils utilized in processed foods (baked items, fried foods).

- Impact: Trans fat improve LDL cholesterol levels and decrease HDL levels of cholesterol, growing the risk of heart disorder. They are also associated with infection and may make a contribution to insulin resistance, that may circuitously have an effect on cancer hazard.

3. Omega6 Fatty Acids

Sources: Found in vegetable oils (corn oil, soybean oil) and processed meals containing those oils.

- Impact: In excess, omega6 fatty acids can promote inflammation, that's connected to persistent diseases consisting of most cancers. Balancing omega6 consumption with omega3 fatty acids (located in fatty fish, flaxseeds) is vital for universal health.

RED AND PROCESSED MEATS

1. Red Meat

Sources: Includes beef, red meat, lamb.

Impact: Consumption of beef, specially processed forms (e.G., sausages, bacon), is related to an increased threat of colorectal most cancers. The mechanisms are not completely understood but may additionally involve the formation of carcinogenic compounds at some point of cooking or processing, and the presence of heme iron.

2. Processed Meats

Sources: Includes bacon, sausages, warm puppies, deli meats.

Impact: Classified as carcinogenic to people (Group 1) by the International Agency for Research on Cancer (IARC). Processed meats incorporate additives and go through renovation techniques (smoking, curing) which could lead to the formation of carcinogenic compounds like nitrosamines.

RECOMMENDATIONS

- Limit Consumption: Reduce intake of saturated fat through deciding on leaner cuts of meat, trimming seen fat, and choosing plant based resources of fat (avocado, nuts, seeds).
- Avoid Trans Fats: Read meals labels and avoid products containing partly

hydrogenated oils. Choose more healthy cooking oils like olive oil or canola oil.

- Moderate Red and Processed Meats: Limit intake of beef and processed meats. Opt for options like rooster, fish, beans, or plant primarily based proteins (tofu, tempeh).

- Balanced Diet: Focus on a balanced eating regimen wealthy in end result, veggies, complete grains, and lean proteins to lessen universal cancer risk and promote lengthy time period health.

- The function of dangerous fat and purple meats in most cancers development

- Unhealthy fats and purple meats had been related to an elevated chance of most cancers improvement, particularly for sure varieties of cancers.

UNHEALTHY FATS

1. Saturated Fats

- Sources: Found frequently in animal products inclusive of beef, complete fat dairy merchandise (butter, cheese), and a few plant oils (coconut oil, palm oil).

- Impact:

- Cardiovascular Health: High consumption of saturated fat is connected to multiplied stages of LDL (horrific) ldl cholesterol and can make contributions to cardiovascular sicknesses.

- Cancer Risk: While proof linking saturated fat at once to most cancers is much less clear than for cardiovascular diseases, some studies advise that a weight reduction plan excessive in saturated fat might also growth the chance of certain cancers, likely via mechanisms related to infection and oxidative stress.

2. Trans Fats

- Sources: Found in partially hydrogenated oils used in processed ingredients (baked goods, fried foods).

Impact:

- Cardiovascular Health: Trans fat increase LDL levels of cholesterol and decrease HDL (properly) levels of cholesterol, growing the chance of heart sickness and stroke.

- Cancer Risk: Consumption of trans fats has been associated with an elevated hazard of cardiovascular sicknesses, however direct evidence linking trans fat to cancer is confined. However, the general inflammatory and metabolic effects of trans fats may indirectly affect cancer chance.

3. Omega6 Fatty Acids

● Sources: Found in vegetable oils (corn oil, soybean oil) and processed meals containing these oils.

● Impact:

● Inflammation: In extra, omega6 fatty acids can sell continual inflammation, that is connected to cancer development and development.

● Balance with Omega3s: Maintaining a balanced ratio of omega6 to omega3 fatty acids is important for typical health. High consumption of omega6 fatty acids relative to omega3s can also make a contribution to inflammation and probably boom most cancers danger.

RED AND PROCESSED MEATS

1. Red Meat

● Sources: Includes beef, beef, lamb.

● Colo rectal Cancer: Consumption of pork, in particular processed

bureaucracy (e.G., sausages, bacon), is
continuously associated with an
expanded risk of colorectal most cancers.

- Possible Mechanisms: Cooking red
  meat at high temperatures or processing
  it could lead to the formation of
  carcinogenic compounds (hetero cyclic
  amines, poly cyclic fragrant
  hydrocarbons) that can harm cells in the
  colon.

2. Processed Meats

Sources: Includes bacon, sausages, hot dogs,
deli meats.

Impact:

- Carcinogenicity: Classified as
  carcinogenic to people (Group 1)
  through the International Agency for
  Research on Cancer (IARC). Processed
  meats contain additives and go through
  upkeep strategies (smoking, curing) that
  may result in the formation of

carcinogenic compounds like nitrosamines.

- Increased Cancer Risk: Consumption of processed meats has been linked to an improved danger of colorectal most cancers, stomach most cancers, and possibly different cancers.

ALCOHOL AND CAFFEINE

Alcohol and caffeine are substances that many humans eat frequently, but their consequences on fitness, along with their capacity function in most cancers development, are crucial concerns.

ALCOHOL

1. Cancer Risk

- Types of Cancer: Alcohol consumption is a acknowledged risk element for several types of cancer, including:
- Breast Cancer: Even moderate alcohol intake has been related to an extended threat of breast most cancers in ladies.

- Liver Cancer: Chronic alcohol intake can lead to liver cirrhosis and boom the hazard of liver most cancers.
- Colorectal Cancer: Higher alcohol consumption is related to an increased chance of colorectal most cancers.

2. Mechanisms

- Ethanol Metabolism: When alcohol is metabolized within the body, it produces acetaldehyde, a poisonous substance that can damage DNA and proteins, potentially leading to most cancers.
- Hormone Levels: Alcohol intake can affect hormone tiers, such as estrogen in ladies, which might also make a contribution to breast cancer chance.
- Nutrient Absorption: Heavy alcohol intake can interfere with the absorption of essential vitamins, which might be vital for average fitness and cancer prevention.

3. Recommendations

● Moderation: To reduce most cancers danger and overall health dangers, it's suggested to restrict alcohol consumption:

● Women: No multiple drink per day.

Men: No more than liquids in step with day.

Abstinence: For individuals at higher risk of alcoholrelated cancers or people with a history of alcohol use disorder, avoiding alcohol altogether is suggested.

CAFFEINE

1. Cancer Risk

● Research Findings: Studies on caffeine intake and cancer danger had been blended, with some suggesting capability protecting outcomes towards certain cancers:

- Skin Cancer: Some studies suggests that caffeine may assist reduce the threat of non melanoma skin cancers.
- Liver Cancer: Some research advise a probable protective impact of coffee consumption against liver most cancers.

2. Mechanisms

- Antioxidant Properties: Caffeine is a robust antioxidant that may neutralize loose radicals, that are implicated in most cancers development.
- Potential Hormonal Effects: Caffeine might also have an effect on hormone ranges, together with cortisol and insulin, which could theoretically have an impact on most cancers danger, but greater research is wanted.

3. Recommendations

- Moderation: For maximum adults, slight caffeine consumption is taken into consideration secure and may even offer some fitness benefits:

- Daily Limits: Generally, up to four hundred milligrams (approximately 4 cups of brewed coffee) in line with day is considered safe for maximum healthful adults.

- Individual Sensitivity: Some individuals can be extra touchy to caffeine and ought to modify their consumption accordingly.

Guidelines on alcohol and caffeine intake Certainly!

ALCOHOL CONSUMPTION GUIDELINES

1. Moderate Drinking Definition

Women: Up to one standard drink according to day.

Men: Up to two widespread beverages consistent with day.

2. What Counts as a Standard Drink?

- Beer: 12 oz (approximately 355 milliliters) of beer with approximately five% alcohol content material.

- Wine: five oz (approximately 148 milliliters) of wine with about 12% alcohol content.

- Liquor/Spirits: 1.5 oz. (approximately 44 milliliters) of distilled spirits with about forty% alcohol content material.

3. Considerations

- Pregnancy: No amount of alcohol is considered secure during being pregnant.

- Health Conditions: Individuals with positive medical situations or taking medicines must talk over with healthcare providers regarding alcohol intake.

- Abstinence: For individuals with a history of alcohol use ailment or the ones at better hazard of alcohol related cancers, abstinence is recommended.

CAFFEINE CONSUMPTION
GUIDELINES

1. Daily Limit

Adults: Up to four hundred milligrams of caffeine in step with day is typically considered secure for most healthy adults.

- Pregnancy: Limited caffeine intake (normally less than 200 milligrams in keeping with day) is recommended in the course of being pregnant to lessen the risk of damaging consequences at the fetus.

2. Sources of Caffeine

- Coffee: Typically consists of eighty100 milligrams of caffeine in line with eight ounce cup.

- Tea: Contains about 3050 milligrams of caffeine according to 8ounce cup, relying on the type and brewing approach.

- Energy Drinks: Can range widely in caffeine content, regularly containing high levels (as much as 300 milligrams or greater according to serving).

3. Considerations

- Individual Sensitivity: Some individuals can be greater sensitive to caffeine and can want to limit their intake as a consequence.

- Health Conditions: People with certain medical conditions (e.G., tension disorders, heart conditions) must display or limit caffeine consumption as suggested through healthcare vendors.

- Timing: Avoid ingesting caffeine close to bedtime to save you sleep disturbances.

CHAPTER 5: SPECIAL CONSIDERATIONS DURING TREATMENT

NUTRITION DURING CHEMOTHERAPY AND RADIATION

DIETARY WISHES AND ADJUSTMENTS IN THE COURSE OF REMEDY

During most cancers remedy, retaining a balanced food plan is vital to aid basic fitness, manipulate side effects, and aid in recuperation.

GENERAL DIETARY GUIDELINES

1. Nutrient Dense Foods

Focus on complete meals which might be rich in vitamins which includes fruits, veggies, complete grains, lean proteins, and wholesome fat.

Choose loads of hues to make certain a large spectrum of vitamins, minerals, and antioxidants.

2. Adequate Protein Intake

Include lean proteins like fowl, fish, beans, lentils, tofu, and eggs to guide muscle maintenance and restore.

3. Healthy Fats

Incorporate assets of wholesome fat inclusive of avocados, nuts, seeds, and olive oil to aid universal fitness and energy levels.

4. Hydration

Drink masses of fluids, especially water, to live hydrated. This is mainly important for the duration of treatments that could cause dehydration or affect kidney function.

5. Fiber Rich Foods

Include fiber from complete grains, fruits, and vegetables to guide digestive health and save you constipation, a not unusual side impact of a few treatments.

ADJUSTMENTS DURING TREATMENT

1. Managing Side Effects

- Nausea: Choose bland, without difficulty digestible foods. Avoid sturdy smelling or greasy foods. Eat small, common food.

- Mouth Sores: Opt for soft, moist ingredients like soups, smoothies, and yogurt. Avoid spicy, acidic, or hard textured meals.

- Fatigue: Eat small food and snacks all through the day to maintain energy levels. Choose ingredients high in complicated carbohydrates for sustained power.

- Changes in Taste: Experiment with seasonings and marinades to beautify flavor. Cold or room temperature meals can be higher tolerated.

Weight Changes: Work with a dietitian to alter calorie consumption based totally on character desires and treatment outcomes.

2. Food Safety

Practice right meals protection measures to reduce the danger of food borne illnesses, mainly if immune function is compromised.

Avoid raw or under cooked meats, fish, and eggs. Wash culmination and vegetables very well.

3. Supplements

Discuss with healthcare vendors before taking any dietary supplements. Some can also interfere with remedies or exacerbate aspect results.

4. Personalized Guidance

Seek steering from a registered dietitian that specialize in oncology to create a customized nutrition plan that meets specific desires for the duration of treatment.

MANAGING SIDE EFFECTS WITH DIET

Managing side results with weight loss plan throughout most cancers remedy is important for keeping nutritional status, dealing with symptoms, and helping average nicely being.

1. Nausea and Vomiting

Dietary Tips:

- Eat small, common meals at some point of the day.
- Opt for bland, low fats, and without difficulty digestible ingredients together with crackers, toast, rice, and boiled potatoes.
- Avoid robust smelling or greasy meals.
- Stay hydrated with clean fluids like water, natural teas, or ginger tea.
- Consider ginger (in tea or as a complement) which can also help alleviate nausea.

2. Mouth Sores and Difficulty Swallowing

Dietary Tips:

- Choose gentle, moist ingredients like soups, smoothies, yogurt, and mashed potatoes.

- Avoid acidic, spicy, or difficult textured foods that could aggravate the mouth.

- Rinse your mouth with a saltwater answer earlier than and after food.

- Use a straw for drinking liquids to skip painful regions in the mouth.

3. Taste Changes (Dysgeusia)

Dietary Tips:

- Experiment with specific flavors and seasonings to find what tastes fine.

- Cold or room temperature ingredients can be greater palatable than warm ingredients.

- Marinate meats or greens to decorate taste.

- Avoid metal utensils if ingredients taste metallic.

4. Fatigue

Dietary Tips:

- Eat small, frequent meals and snacks at some point of the day to maintain energy ranges.

- Include complex carbohydrates together with complete grains, fruits, and vegetables to offer sustained electricity.

- Limit caffeine intake, specially later inside the day, to avoid disrupting sleep patterns.

5. Constipation

Dietary Tips:

Increase fiber intake gradually from end result, veggies, whole grains, and legumes.

- Stay hydrated with the aid of consuming lots of fluids, specifically water.

- Include ingredients with natural laxative residences including prunes, figs, and bran cereals.

- Engage in mild physical activity if possible, as it may assist stimulate bowel movements.

6. Diarrhea

Dietary Tips:

- Avoid excessive fiber meals, greasy or fried ingredients, highly spiced meals, and dairy merchandise.

- Opt for low fiber meals along with bananas, white rice, applesauce, and toast (BRAT diet).

- Drink masses of fluids to live hydrated and update electrolytes if needed (e.G., with sports beverages or electrolyte solutions).

7. Changes in Appetite and Weight Loss

Dietary Tips:

- Eat small, nutrient dense food and snacks at some stage in the day.

- Choose excessive calorie, excessive protein ingredients consisting of nuts, seeds, nut butters, cheese, and yogurt.

- Add healthful fat like avocado, olive oil, and fatty fish to food to growth calorie intake.

- Consider nutritional supplements as advocated by means of healthcare carriers.

FOODS AND STRATEGIES TO RELIEVE REMEDY SIDE EFFECTS

During most cancers remedy, various side results can effect urge for food, digestion, and common nicely being. 1. Nausea and Vomiting

- Ginger: Known for its antinausea properties, ginger can be consumed as tea, grated fresh into hot water, or in ginger sweets.

- Peppermint: Peppermint tea or sucking on peppermint chocolates can assist soothe the stomach.
- Plain Crackers or Toast: These bland, low fat options can ease nausea.
- Clear Liquids: Stay hydrated with clean fluids like water, herbal teas, or electrolyte answers.

Avoid Strong Odors: Steer clear of sturdy smelling foods or cooking odors that can trigger nausea.

2. Mouth Sores and Difficulty Swallowing

- Soft Foods: Opt for smoothies, yogurt, applesauce, mashed potatoes, and soups.
- Cold Foods: Foods served cold or at room temperature may be greater soothing.

- Avoid Acidic Foods: Skip citrus end result, tomatoes, and spicy ingredients which can irritate sores.

- Gentle Mouth Care: Rinse with saltwater or a baking soda solution to maintain the mouth clean and decrease infection.

3. Taste Changes (Dysgeusia)

- Strong Flavors: Experiment with more potent flavors and spices to decorate flavor perception.

- Marinades and Sauces: Use flavorful marinades or sauces to enhance the taste of meats and veggies.

- Citrus Fruits: Some humans find that citrus end result or bitter chocolates can temporarily improve flavor sensitivity.

4. Fatigue

- Complex Carbohydrates: Choose complete grains, end result, and greens for sustained energy.

- Small, Frequent Meals: Eating smaller food during the day can help maintain power stages.

- Hydration: Drink lots of water to stay hydrated, which could reduce feelings of fatigue.

5. Constipation

- High Fiber Foods: Gradually introduce fiber wealthy ingredients like complete grains, culmination (with skins), and vegetables.

- Prunes and Fig Compote: These natural laxatives can assist alter bowel moves.

- Fluid Intake: Drink masses of water and herbal teas to soften stools and promote regularity.

6. Diarrhea

- BRAT Diet: Stick to bananas, rice, applesauce, and toast to assist company stools and decrease irritation.

- Avoid High Fiber Foods: Steer clean of uncooked vegetables, whole grains, and spicy foods that can irritate diarrhea.

- Hydration: Drink electrolyte solutions or sports activities beverages to update lost fluids and minerals.

7. Changes in Appetite and Weight Loss

- High Calorie, Nutrient Dense Foods: Include nuts, seeds, avocados, cheese, and complete fats yogurt to boom calorie consumption.

- Small, Frequent Meals: Eating smaller, more frequent meals can be less overwhelming and extra practicable.

- Protein Rich Foods: Lean meats, fish, eggs, and legumes provide essential vitamins and sell satiety.

SUPPLEMENTS AND HERBAL REMEDIES

Supplements and herbal remedies are frequently considered as complementary strategies to help health for the duration of cancer treatment. It's crucial to technique their use with caution and underneath the guidance of healthcare providers, as some dietary supplements may additionally have interaction with remedies or medicines.

Supplements

1. Multivitamins

Purpose: Provide various vitamins and minerals to help overall dietary consumption.

Considerations: Choose dietary supplements especially formulated for cancer sufferers, as they'll have adjusted degrees of sure vitamins.

2. Omega3 Fatty Acids

- Purpose: Support coronary heart fitness and can help lessen irritation.

- Sources: Fish oil supplements or plant primarily based assets like flaxseed oil.

- Considerations: Consult with healthcare vendors, as omegathree supplements can have an effect on blood clotting and engage with sure medicines.

3. Probiotics

Purpose: Promote gut health and resource in digestion.

Sources: Supplements containing useful bacteria lines like Lactobacillus and Bifidobacterium.

Considerations: Helpful for handling digestive issues, however discuss with healthcare carriers, particularly if undergoing remedies that affect the immune system.

4. Vitamin D

Purpose: Support bone fitness and immune function.

Sources: Supplements or fortified ingredients.

Considerations: Levels may additionally need tracking, in particular if sunlight publicity is restrained or throughout certain treatments.

5. Herbal Supplements

Purpose: Some herbs like turmeric (curcumin), green tea extract, or ginger may additionally have antioxidant or anti inflammatory houses.

Considerations: Discuss with healthcare carriers due to capability interactions with treatments and varying degrees of evidence supporting their use.

HERBAL REMEDIES

1. Ginger

Purpose: Known for its antinausea houses.

Forms: Fresh ginger, ginger tea, or supplements.

Considerations: Generally safe, but talk over with healthcare providers, especially if taking blood thinning medicinal drugs.

2. Turmeric (Curcumin)

Purpose: Has anti inflammatory homes.

Forms: Turmeric spice or curcumin supplements.

Considerations: May engage with sure medications; discuss with healthcare carriers.

3. Green Tea Extract

Purpose: Contains antioxidants (catechins) that may have fitness benefits.

Considerations: Contains caffeine and might interact with medications; use cautiously below healthcare provider steerage.

SAFE USE OF DIETARY SUPPLEMENTS AND NATURAL TREATMENTS

Using dietary supplements and natural remedies competently, in particular at some stage in most cancers treatment, calls for careful attention and consultation with healthcare companies.

1. Consult Healthcare Providers

Always Consult: Before beginning any supplement or herbal remedy, discuss it together with your oncologist, primary care health practitioner, or a registered dietitian who specializes in oncology.

Medical History: Inform them about your scientific records, along with cutting edge remedies, medicinal drugs (prescription and over the counter), allergic reactions, and any prepresent situations.

2. Choose Reputable Sources

 Quality Assurance: Select supplements from authentic manufacturers that adhere to right production practices (GMP) and feature gone through third birthday celebration trying out for purity and potency.

 3. Consider Potential Interactions

- Medication Interactions: Some dietary supplements can engage with cancer treatments, lowering their effectiveness or inflicting negative consequences. Examples include:

- Antioxidants: High doses may additionally interfere with chemotherapy or radiation therapy.

- Herbal Supplements: Ginger, turmeric, and inexperienced tea extract can have interaction with medications; talk their use with healthcare providers.

4. Monitor for Side Effects

 Be Vigilant: Watch for any facet consequences or destructive reactions whilst beginning a brand new supplement or natural remedy.

 Report Changes: Promptly document any new signs and symptoms or changes in fitness to your healthcare group.

5. Follow Recommended Dosages

- Dosage Instructions: Adhere strictly to recommended dosages supplied via healthcare companies or as indicated on the complement label.

- Avoid Overdose: More isn't always necessarily better; excessive doses can be dangerous.

6. Be Cautious During Treatments

Timing: Avoid taking supplements close to chemotherapy or radiation remedy classes unless permitted through healthcare companies.

Immune Function: Be cautious with dietary supplements which could affect immune characteristic, specially if present process remedies that suppress the immune system.

7. Inform Healthcare Providers

Open Communication: Keep healthcare vendors informed about all dietary supplements and natural treatments you take, consisting of dosages and frequency.

Integration into Care: Supplements ought to complement, no longer update, conventional medical remedies.

8. Consider Nutritional Needs

Focus on Nutrition: Emphasize a well balanced diet rich in end result, veggies, whole grains, lean proteins, and healthful fats as the inspiration of your nutritional support.